FAST LIKE NEVER BEFORE

Unlock Your Potential to Burn Fat, Balance Hormones, and Fuel Your Soul with Spiritual Strength!

DEREK HEATON

BOOKS BY THE AUTHOR

QUITTING MADE EASY

SOBER REFLECTIONS

DEFEATING ANXIETY

"EVERYONE CAN PERFORM MAGIC,
EVERYONE CAN REACH HIS GOAL, IF
HE IS ABLE TO THINK, IF HE IS ABLE
TO WAIT, IF HE IS ABLE TO FAST!!'

-Hermann Hesse

TABLE OF CONTENTS

"EVERYONE CAN PERFORM MAGIC, EVERYONE CAN REACH HIS GOAL, IF HE IS ABLE TO THINK, IF HE IS ABLE TO WAIT, IF HE IS ABLE TO FAST!!'

-Hermann Hesse

TABLE OF CONTENTS

Introduction

Fast food and continual exercise seem to be the norm in our fast-paced modern life, but we sometimes forget about the power of fasting as a crucial component of health and well-being. For a moment, try to picture your body as a well-oiled machine that, like all machines, occasionally requires maintenance and rest to function at its peak. Here's where fasting becomes relevant.

Fundamentally, fasting is an age-old custom that brings simplicity to an increasingly complicated society. It's about revival, revitalization, and rejuvenation—not about hardship or deprivation. We're going to go on a life-changing adventure together in the upcoming chapters, one that will reveal the tricks of using fasting to burn fat, boost energy, and realign your body's complex hormonal balance.

We are going to learn that fasting is much more than just not eating; it is a deep state of healing. It's similar to restarting your smartphone when it gets slow—it's like pressing the reset button on your body's metabolism. This is about reconnecting with your body's intrinsic knowledge, not about crash diets or unsustainable habits.

Think of your body as an experienced gardener. Your body needs times of fasting to thrive, just as a garden needs trimming and rest to produce the most exquisite and abundant blooms. We shall demystify the science of fasting throughout this book and provide you with plain, understandable reasons. Consider it as unlocking the guidebook for the best possible functioning of your body.

However, this trip is about the genuine, accessible stories of people who have used fasting's healing power to change their lives, not just statistics and numbers. We'll relate anecdotes and comparisons from ordinary life to help make the body's experience of fasting more relatable.

We will address your 30-day fasting journey day by day as we go along, providing you with the resources, information, and motivation you need to start along this incredibly transforming path. It's like having a helpful guide stroll beside you while you negotiate the challenging landscape of fasting.

This is your chance to rediscover the simplicity and purity of a practice that has been a part of human history for generations and to re-establish a connection with the intrinsic wisdom of your body. By doing this, you will experience a greater sense of vitality and well-being in addition to burning fat, increasing your energy, and balancing your hormones. This is the start of a journey that will change the way you think about food, your body, and your overall health.

So buckle up, fellow wellness seeker, and join me as we set out on an enlightening 30-day adventure to discover the amazing possibilities that fasting has to offer. Prepare to be amazed by your body's incredible ability to recover and thrive as we examine how fasting can transform fat-burning, increase energy, and balance hormones.

SECTION I

CHAPTER I

THE SCIENCE OF FASTING: A BASIC UNDERSTANDING

Fasting is a natural condition that your body enters when you refrain from eating for a set amount of time; it's not a magical or difficult concept. The science of fasting will be dissected in this chapter, with simple language and analogies to make it seem as natural as breathing.

The Energy Stores in the Body: A Comparison with Savings Accounts

Consider your energy stores as a savings account and your body as a financial institution. Your body starts to take energy (calories) out of this account when you fast. Energy is deposited into this account when you eat. When you go without food, your body uses its stored energy, much as you could use your savings to cover unforeseen costs.

Glucagon and Insulin: The Blood Sugar Regulators

To comprehend the impact of fasting on your body's energy equilibrium, let's talk about the functions of insulin and glucagon. Together, these hormones function as a dynamic combination to keep your blood sugar levels stable.

Insulin functions as a key that opens your cells' doors to let glucose, or sugar, in. When you consume, it aids in the storage of surplus energy as fat.

Conversely, glucagon functions similarly to insulin in the opposite way. Glucagon signals your body to release stored energy, mostly from fat cells, when you're fasting or need additional energy.

Think of insulin as the key that keeps the goods (glucose) hidden in the pantry of your body. Glucagon is the key that lets you access the groceries for energy when you're fasting.

The Body's Savings Account Withdrawal in Fat-Burning Mode

Your body's principal objective during a fast is to keep you supplied with energy at all times. It starts burning fat for fuel as soon as the easily available glucose is exhausted. This shift is analogous to spending the money in your savings account (fat) instead of the cash in your wallet (glucose).

In other words, when you start a fast, you're instructing your body to start burning the fat that has been stored for a rainy day.

Hormones and Cell Repair: The Remediation Team of the Body

Fasting provides your body with much-needed housekeeping time in addition to energy. It triggers procedures like autophagy, which allows your cells to recycle and remove damaged parts. This is similar to organizing your closet to get rid of outdated, worn-out clothes and make room for new, useful ones.

To put it briefly, the science of fasting entails a careful balancing act between energy storage and utilization. When you fast, your body mobilizes its stores of energy, mostly fat, to sustain you and launches a cellular cleanup crew for upkeep.

The basis for your 30-day fasting experience is this chapter. Comprehending these fundamentals is akin to possessing the keys to a treasure trove of health advantages. We'll look at how to apply this information to successfully burn fat, increase energy, and balance hormones in the next chapters.

CHAPTER 2

BREAKING YOUR FAST, A SAFE TRANSITION

Breaking your fast is an important step in which you should reintroduce nutrients to your body gradually and thoughtfully. This comprehensive guide will help to ensure a healthy and safe transition:

1. Start with Hydration: Fill your body back up with water first. To help your digestive system and replenish fluids, drink herbal teas or water.

Hydration functions similarly to prime soil for new growth.

2. Choose Light Foods: Include foods that are simple to digest and light, like fruits and vegetables. They are your garden's first sprouts, breaking the ground ready for larger, more substantial nutrients.

3. Include Good Fats: To provide long-lasting energy, include foods high in healthy fats, such as nuts or avocados. Consider these to be the sturdy leaves that give your garden structure and depth.

4. Gradual Protein Intake: Reintroduce proteins gradually, beginning with lean foods like legumes or chicken. This is like adding strong branches to your already-thriving garden.

5. Watch Portion Sizes: Give your stomach time to acclimate to the larger volume by being mindful of portion sizes. It's similar to carefully calculating how much fertilizer to use in your garden to ensure maximum growth.

6. Listen to Your Body: Observe closely how each food group makes you feel. Pay attention to your body's signals for the best nutrition, just as you would watch how plants react to various nutrients.

7. Think About Nutrient Density: Select foods high in vitamins and minerals that are high in nutrients. It's similar to choosing high-quality soil for your garden and guaranteeing a rich base for long-term well-being.

Safely breaking your fast is akin to creating a nutritional symphony for your body. You can give your digestive system the time and encouragement it needs to reawaken and flourish by taking this methodical approach. Breaking your fast becomes a harmonious process that creates the conditions for ongoing health and vitality, much like taking care of a flourishing garden.

CHAPTER 3

SUCCESSFUL RECIPES FOR FASTING

- *Quick and Nutrient-Rich Breakfast Smoothie*

Ingredients

Berries: Rich in antioxidants, berries enhance flavor and improve general health.

Spinach: Rich in minerals and vitamins, spinach boosts nutrition without adding too many calories.

Greek Yogurt: Greek yogurt is a high-protein food that helps you feel content and full.

Almond milk is a dairy-free substitute that has the same creamy feel as conventional milk but without the added calories.

Chia seeds: Packed full of fiber and good fats, these little powerhouses provide you with long-lasting energy.

This is a simple, fast-preparing, high-nutrient morning smoothie that is suitable for fasting. Berries have a tangy and sweet taste and are packed with antioxidants that are good for the whole body. Without providing many calories, spinach contributes vitamins and minerals. In addition to adding to the smoothie's smoothness, Greek yogurt increases its protein level, which aids in maintaining muscle mass when fasting. A dairy-free liquid foundation is offered by almond milk, while chia seeds add fiber and good fats that help you feel full all morning.

- *Grilled Chicken Salad with Avocado Dressing*

Ingredients

Grilled chicken is a lean protein that keeps you full and helps maintain the health of your muscles.

Mixed Greens: Adding a range of leafy greens to the salad increases its vitamin, mineral, and fiber content.

Cherry Tomatoes: Packed with antioxidants and taste.

Cucumber: Increases hydration and adds a cool crunch.

Avocado Dressing: A nutritious and creamy dressing with good fats derived from avocados.

For lunch or dinner, this grilled chicken salad is a filling and well-balanced choice. Lean protein sources like grilled chicken are crucial for preserving muscle mass during fasting. While cherry tomatoes and cucumbers give freshness and moisture, mixed greens provide a range of vitamins and minerals. In addition to adding taste to the salad, the avocado dressing offers heart-healthy lipids. This salad's protein, fiber, and healthy fats all work together to promote satiety, which makes it a fantastic option for a satisfying and fast-friendly supper.

- *Grilled chicken with mango and avocado salad*

Ingredients

The lean protein source is grilled chicken breast.

Ripe Mango: Contributes vitamins and natural sweetness.

Avocado: Offers a creamy mouthfeel and good fats.

Mixed greens: Rich in fiber and antioxidants, such as spinach and arugula.

Lime vinaigrette: a zesty dressing made with lime juice, olive oil, and a hint of honey.

Getting ready:

1. Cook the chicken breast completely on the grill.
2. Chop the avocado and mango into small pieces.
3. Combine avocado, mango, and mixed greens in a bowl.
4. Arrange the grilled chicken slices over the salad.
5. Add a lime vinaigrette drizzle and gently stir.

The grilled chicken, avocado, and juicy mango provide a healthy dose of protein, fat, and natural sweetness in this colorful salad. On non-fasting days, the mixed greens add vital nutrients and make a vibrant, tasty salad. The lime vinaigrette improves the flavor and nutritional profile while adding a refreshing element.

- *Lentil Soup for Vegetarians*

Ingredients

Lentils: A great source of fiber and plant-based protein.

Carrots, celery, and onion: To create a savory vegetable foundation.

Depth of taste is provided by vegetable broth.

Turmeric, cumin, and garlic are seasonings with anti-inflammatory and flavorful qualities.

Getting ready:

1. Garlic, onions, carrots, and celery should be sautéed until tender.
2. Stir in spices, lentils, and vegetable broth.
3. Once the lentils are soft, simmer them.
4. Serve hot, adding seasoning to taste.

On non-fasting days, this filling and healthy lentil soup is a great choice for vegetarians. The flavor profile is enhanced by the addition of veggies and spices, and lentils provide plant-based protein and fiber. Not only is the soup filling, but it's also a terrific method to get those important elements into your diet.

CHAPTER 4

WHAT TO EAT WHEN FASTING

Water

water is not food, right? Is it? However, it is an essential component to get you through your intermittent fasting. Your body uses glycogen—a type of sugar stored in your liver—when you fast for sixteen hours. Your energy is expended and electrolytes are used when you fast. Therefore, it becomes essential to maintain proper hydration.

However, several factors, including weight, sex, and age, affect how much water you should drink. Experts advise adults to consume eight glasses of water or more each day. Water consumption improves blood flow and keeps you from being dehydrated. Several health problems, including lethargy, nausea, weight gain, and exhaustion, are associated with dehydration.

One useful indicator of dehydration is the color of your urine. Urine should typically be a light yellow color; if it's dark yellow, your body is becoming dehydrated.

Foods with Added Salt

You could discover that you require more salt in your diet than usual while fasting. When fasting, make sure to season your food with salt. It's also a good idea to take an electrolyte supplement if necessary.

Eggs

Eggs are a fantastic fast-food option!

The ideal superfood is this one! The harmony of lipids, proteins, and amino acids makes it almost the ideal diet found in nature! The eggs are quick to prepare and packed with protein. It is advised that you incorporate eggs into your intermittent diet as they provide you the essential nutrients and help you feel satisfied.

Cruciferous Vegetables

Broccoli, cabbage, cauliflower, and Brussels sprouts are among the greatest vegetables to eat intermittently rapidly. They have a ton of fiber. It's crucial to eat extra fiber when you eat seldom to prevent constipation.

In addition to being high in minerals, vitamins C, E, and K, and antioxidant activity, cruciferous vegetables are also rich in beta-carotene. Numerous studies indicate that the antioxidant activity of these veggies may help prevent cancer.

They help you feel satisfied so that you can fast for a longer period.

Avocado

Avocado is a fantastic food for fasting and has healthy fasts!

A nutrient-dense, whole-food option that lowers your risk of obesity and prevents weight gain is avocado. Fruits with a medium calorie count, and avocados aid in the reduction of obesity. It has nutrients such as fiber, phytochemicals, and monounsaturated fatty acids (MUFAs).

Avocado's dietary fiber improves satiety and blocks the absorption of fat, which helps to prevent weight gain.

Avocados are a great source of monounsaturated fatty acids (MUFAs), which can help reduce extra body fat and prevent weight gain. After a period of fasting, healthy fats are required.

Avocados have been shown to increase fullness, decrease appetite, and reduce food intake. Additionally, avocados affect gut hormones, which may help you control your calorie intake and weight in the long run.

Seafood

The Dietary Guidelines for Americans recommend that you eat at least two to three servings of fish per week, weighing between two and three ounces. Fish, prawns, and shrimp are examples of seafood that is high in protein, vitamin D, and good fats. Because it is high in nutrients and low in harmful calories, seafood is a great option for fasting. Aim for salmon and other smaller fish instead of mercury-rich fish.

Fish eating is thought to be beneficial and may lower the risk of cardiovascular disease. Fish is something you should include in your intermittent fasting diet.

Grass- Fed Meats

Try to eat only grass-fed and grass-finished red meats when you consume them. Throughout their lives, cows who are fed grass produce meat that is higher in nutrients and hence healthier. When choosing the appropriate cuts, this is packed with healthy fats. Try to include as much leaner ground beef as possible (85%–15%), ribeye steaks, NY Strip, ground lamb, ground lamb chops, venison, elk, bison, and other wild game in your diet. The liver, kidney, and heart are among the superfoods found in nature that are packed with vitamins and other nutrients, provided you can consume them.

Legumes

You need to include some low-calorie carbohydrates in your diet because foods high in carbohydrates provide you with energy for your everyday activities. Low-calorie carbohydrates high in vitamins and proteins include legumes and beans.

Beans and legumes help you feel satisfied while you're fasting. Research indicates consuming legumes, chickpeas, black beans, and peas is associated with a reduction in body weight even in the absence of calorie restriction.

Potatoes

Potatoes are on the list of the best meals to fast!

White potatoes are an excellent addition to your intermittent fasting food plan because they are quickly absorbed. Taken with a source of protein, it's the ideal post-workout snack. Your muscles' energy can be replenished by it. Potato starch is beneficial to the intestinal flora.

Berries and Fruits

Berries and fruits are high in carotenoids, vitamins, and minerals and are considered healthful. We recommend that you start your day with a dish full of mixed fruits and berries. You feel satiated and well after eating these fruits. Consuming 400g or more of fruits and vegetables each day is advised.

Fruits facilitate smooth digestion by aiding in the breakdown of proteins. They also lead to weight loss, less cell damage, and better skin health.

Nuts

Because they contain healthy fats, you can incorporate a variety of nuts into your diet. When you have a craving for food during your intermittent fast, these are great options. Numerous studies indicate that eating nuts lowers the risk of death, type 2 diabetes, and cardiovascular diseases.

If you don't have gluten sensitivity, only eat whole grains; otherwise, stay away

Because whole grains are high in natural fiber, they can help you feel fuller and keep your weight stable. Whole grains encompass buckwheat, brown rice, cracked wheat, millets, oats, whole wheat bread, and pasta.

There is evidence connecting whole grains to a lower risk of diabetes, heart disease, some types of cancer, and other illnesses.

Probiotics

Adding a probiotic drink to your intermittent fasting regimen is a smart idea. It supports healthy gut flora and facilitates improved digestion.

Research indicates that probiotics may lessen irritable bowel syndrome and assist in balancing the amounts of beneficial bacteria in your digestive system.

Probiotics during intermittent fasting have been shown in another study to enhance glucose tolerance, aid in weight loss, and improve glycemic control in prediabetes.

Smoothies

Smoothies with peanut butter, avocado, berries, bananas, and dried fruit can assist you in achieving your nutrient needs. Smoothies that are high in nutrients and health can help you feel full. They enrich your diet with a wealth of vitamins, minerals, and proteins.

You may also include sugar-free fresh fruit juice in your diet; it's full of nutrients and aids in weight loss. Just keep in mind that you should only drink juice during your mealtime. Stick to non-caloric drinks like water, black coffee, or plain tea during the fasting window.

FOODS TO AVOID WHEN FASTING

Certain items must be avoided during fasting to keep a healthy, balanced diet and way of life. Burgers, fries, and nuggets are examples of processed foods that are heavy in calories and can make you crave more food. These foods have empty calories, added sugar, and fat.

The following is a list of foods you should not eat when you are fasting

1. Snacks like fried chips
2. Sugary beverages such as coffee, cold coffee, and carbonated drinks

3. Packaged and processed juices

4. Ice cream and cakes

5. Processed foods—meat, cheese, and the like.

6. Popcorn

7. Candies

8. Carbonated drinks and processed foods have been linked to weight increase in numerous studies. Fresh juices can take the place of fizzy drinks, and salads can be a nutritious substitute for fried items. To maximize the benefits of your intermittent fasting, choose your meals more carefully.

CHAPTER 5

ADVICE AND STRATEGIES FOR A FRUITFUL 30 DAYS FAST

It is made to enhance and assist your fasting journey. Consider it an assortment of useful tactics and perspectives to assist you in overcoming obstacles and optimizing your 30-day fasting experience. Here's a thorough explanation:

1. Strategies for Hydration

Regular Water Consumption: It's important to stay hydrated. Drink water all day long, but especially when you're fasting.

Infuse with Flavor: For a cool twist, infuse your water with a dash of mint or a splash of citrus.

Herbal Teas: To vary your fluid consumption, use herbal teas that aren't caffeine-infused.

2. Ethical Eating on Days Without Fasting

Emphasize Whole Foods High in Vitamins, Minerals, and Fiber to Emphasize Nutrient-Dense Foods.

Include Lean Proteins: To promote muscular health and fullness, include lean proteins in your diet.

Healthy Fats: For long-lasting energy, include foods high in healthy fats, including almonds or avocados.

3. Conscious Eating Techniques

Eat Slowly: To improve digestion and enjoyment, chew your food well and enjoy every bite.

Listen to Your Body: Recognize when you are hungry and full to prevent overindulging.

Practice Gratitude: You can foster a healthy relationship with food by showing thankfulness for every meal.

4. Planning and Preparing Meals

Make a plan: Write down your weekly meal plan, taking into account diversity and a healthy balance of nutrients.

Batch cooking: Make bigger batches of food and portion it out so that it will be convenient to eat on fasting days.

Easy Recipes: Select recipes that are easy to follow, suit your tastes, and are pleasurable to prepare.

5. Handling Cravings and Hunger

Keep Busy: Read, take a stroll, or work on a hobby as ways to divert your attention from hunger.

Hydrate Wisely: To help suppress appetite, sip water when cravings arise.

Mindful Snacking: To fill the time between meals, if necessary, select nutritious snacks such as fruits or nuts.

6. Getting Used to Fasting Schedules

Gradual Introductions: Increase the length of your fasts progressively to ease yourself into it.

Find Your Rhythm: Figure out when to fast based on your energy levels and lifestyle.

Flexibility: Be willing to modify your fasting plan in response to your body's needs.

7. Making Self-Care a Priority

Sufficient Sleep: To maintain general well-being, make sure you obtain a sufficient amount of good sleep.

Mindfulness Practices: To reduce stress, incorporate mindfulness exercises like deep breathing or meditation.

Frequent Exercise: Exercise frequently to improve your mood and energy levels.

8. Tracking Development and Honoring Milestones

Track Your Progress: Maintain a journal to document your

accomplishments and to document your mental and physical well-being.

Celebrate Milestones: Throughout the 30-day journey, give little victories recognition and celebration.

Recall that these pointers are adaptable and can be changed to suit your unique needs and tastes. The secret is to design a fun and lasting fasting experience that supports your overall health objectives.

CHAPTER 6

OBSTACLES AND HOW TO OVERCOME THEM

There are a lot of obstacles to overcome while embarking on a 30-day fast, but you can do it with the correct tactics. Let's examine some typical problems and workable solutions for them:

1. Hunger & Cravings

The difficulty is experiencing strong hunger pangs or desires when fasting.

Answer

Keep Hydrated: To help suppress appetite, sip water, herbal tea, or black coffee.

Select Satisfying Foods: To increase fullness during non-fasting periods, choose lean meats and high-fiber foods.

2. Tiredness and Low Vitality

Difficulty: Being tired, particularly in the early days of the fast.

Answer

Balanced Nutrition: For long-lasting energy, make sure your non-fasting days consist of a well-balanced combination of macronutrients.

Sufficient Rest: To maintain your general energy levels, give good sleep priority.

3. Social Coercion

Difficulty: Handling social settings where food is the main topic.

Answer

Talk to your loved ones about your intention to fast to get their support.

4. Emotive Consumption

Challenge: Relying on food to relieve stress or pass the time when bored.

Answer

Mindfulness Techniques: Use mindfulness exercises to increase your awareness of emotional cues.

Different Coping Mechanisms: Create different coping techniques like writing, meditation, or quick walks.

5. Respect for the Fasting Schedule

The challenge is to follow the selected fasting regimen consistently.

Answer

Flexibility: Allow yourself to modify your fasting window according to your daily schedule and level of energy.

Modest Adjustments: If necessary, progressively lengthen the length of your fasting intervals.

6. Deficit in Nutrients

Difficulty: Worries about getting enough nutrients while fasting.

Answer

Diverse Diet: Make sure you eat a range of nutrient-dense foods on the days you aren't fasting.

Supplementation: To find out if you need to take supplements, speak with a medical practitioner.

6. Idleness or Stagnation

Challenge: Being disinterested in the meals or the schedule.

Answer

Recipe Exploration: To keep dinners interesting, try out different recipes and food pairings.

Intermittent Feasting: To break up the routine, throw in an occasional extra decadent meal.

8. Standstill or Sluggish Progress

Problem: Not achieving the intended outcomes or reaching a weight-loss plateau.

Answer

Evaluate Habits: To find places for improvement, reevaluate your eating and lifestyle choices.

Consult a specialist: To modify your strategy, get advice from a nutritionist or other medical specialist.

It will take a combination of realistic tactics, flexibility, and an optimistic outlook to overcome these obstacles. It's critical to pay attention to your body, adjust as necessary, and acknowledge and appreciate your development as you go. Keep in mind that each person's journey is different, and the secret to having a successful 30-

day fast is figuring out what works best

for you.

63

SECTION II

CHAPTER 7

GETTING READY FOR YOUR 30-DAY FASTING EXPERIENCE

Consider the duration of your 30-day fasting as a road trip. You wouldn't go on a long journey without adequate planning before you left, would you? This also holds for fasting. It is imperative to prepare for this life-changing experience to guarantee a successful and seamless outcome.

Clearly Defined Objectives: Your Pathway

A road trip usually has a destination in mind when it is planned. Fasting is no different. What objectives do you have for the next thirty days? Are you trying to get back into energy, regulate your hormones, or lose a certain amount of weight? Clearly define your goals because they will serve as your guide and roadmap for the trip.

Fasting Kit: The Must-Have Items

Put together your fasting toolkit, just as you wouldn't go on a road trip without carrying the essentials. This entails learning about the different kinds of fasting you'll be performing (water fasting, intermittent fasting, etc.), obtaining recipes and meal plans, and making sure you have any vitamins or supplements you need.

Learning for Yourself: The Road Map

Think of your understanding of fasting as your journey's GPS. Learning about the ins and outs of fasting is crucial. Recognize the various forms of fasting, their mechanisms, and any obstacles you may encounter. You will be guided by this information and assured of staying on the correct path.

Seeking Medical Advice: The Safety Verification

It's similar to having your automobile checked out by a mechanic before you go out on your journey. Seeking advice from your healthcare professional is essential, particularly if you have underlying medical concerns. They can offer tailored guidance to make sure your fasting experience is secure and appropriate for your particular circumstances.

Building a Network of Support: Your Journey Partners

Similar to how you might bring friends or family along for support on a road trip, having a network of support during a fast can be quite beneficial. Having people who support and comprehend your journey, whether they be friends, family, or an online group, may be tremendously beneficial.

Recognizing Difficulties: Expecting Obstacles

You prepare for probable barriers during a road trip, such as traffic, detours, or poor weather. There may be difficulties with fasting as well, such as cravings or hunger sensations. Acquiring the ability to overcome these obstacles is crucial. Consider these obstacles to be overcome on your fasting journey, and we'll offer solutions.

The Pre-Journey Inspection is the Last Check

Usually, you give your car one more inspection before you drive off. In a similar vein, it's a good idea to assess your readiness before the trip. Make sure everything is in order by double-checking your information, your fasting tools, and your support network.

We'll go into more detail about each of these components in this chapter, along with some helpful tips and real-world examples to make sure you're ready for your 30-day fast. A well-prepared faster is more likely to experience the life-changing benefits of fasting, just as a well-prepared traveler is more likely to enjoy a road trip.

CHAPTER 8

BEGINNING YOUR FASTING JOURNEY

---Day 1---

The Start of Your Adventure

Imagine yourself as the lead character in a brand-new chapter of your life on the first day of your fast. You're venturing into uncharted territory, and although there might be doubts, there's also the potential for development and adjustment. Like the opening scene of a movie, this day determines the overall tone of your fasting experience.

Getting Ready: Establishing the Scene

It's important to be ready before you formally start your fast. Consider the first day as setting the scene, like a director setting up props and actors for a performance.

What You Can Do on the First Day

Last Meal: Following a filling last meal, begin your fasting adventure. This aids in psyching you up for the upcoming sprint. The ideal supper is something substantial and well-balanced, like a plate of grilled chicken and veggies.

Hydration: Have a glass of water to start your day. Staying hydrated is essential during your fast. For extra taste, you can even include a slice of lemon.

Mindfulness: Give yourself some time to think. Consider the objectives you have for this 30-day trip. Envision yourself succeeding and reaping the rewards.

Clear Schedule: Try to arrange a day that involves less strenuous tasks. By doing this, you'll be able to lower your stress level and concentrate on enjoying your fast. It's similar to making sure you have a free evening for a noteworthy occasion.

Support System: Share your fasting journey with your support network. Their support, whether from friends, family, or an online group, can be priceless.

Managing Cravings

As Day 1 goes on, you may begin to experience hunger pangs. These are similar to ambient sounds, such as the far-off clamor of a building site while you go about your daily business. You should anticipate them, and keep in mind that they will subside as your body gets used to the fast.

Activities and Distractions

Taking part in activities can assist in diverting your attention from hunger. Think of engaging in a pastime, taking a leisurely walk, or reading a fantastic book. It's similar to focusing on an engrossing film to take your mind off the outer world.

Finishing Up for Day 1

You've done a great job setting the foundation for your fasting journey as Day 1 draws to an end. It feels like the start of a great journey that you have embarked upon by taking this initial step towards well-being. You've got your journey started on the right foot by doing pleasant activities, staying hydrated, and practicing mindfulness.

You will build upon this foundation in the days ahead, and we will support you as you navigate the difficulties and successes of your 30-day fast. your is your first day on your life-changing adventure, and the days ahead will be built on your dedication and readiness.

---Day 2-3---

Entering a state of ketosis

On Days 2 and 3, there is a noticeable change in your physique. It's similar to changing gears on a bike to go from riding a flat stretch of road to climbing a steep hill. Your body starts to shift into a state known as ketosis, in which it mostly uses fat stores rather than glucose for energy. Here are some expectations and actions you can take:

Comprehending Ketosis: The Phase of Fat Burning

Imagine ketosis as the fat-burning catalyst for your fasting expedition.

Your body begins converting fat that has been stored into molecules your body may utilize as fuel, called ketones. Your body converts from utilizing glucose to ketones, just like a hybrid automobile does from using gasoline to electricity.

Physical Changes: Increased Vitality and Mental Sharpness

Your energy levels should start to rise around Days 2-3. This is comparable to how it feels to reach the top of a difficult hill while riding a bike. Your mental clarity and focus will enhance as your body adjusts to ketosis. It may feel as though you've given your body premium gasoline and it's operating at peak efficiency.

Things to Do on Days 2-3

Light Exercise: Your body might enter ketosis more quickly if you engage in light exercise. It is similar to pushing a bike uphill. Try some stretching exercises, yoga, or a stroll. This can help with energy expenditure and speed up the shift.

Maintain Your Hydration: Keep downing large amounts of water. For the ketosis process to occur, proper hydration is necessary. It's similar to making sure the tires on your bike are properly filled for a smoother ride.

Remain Mindful: Engage in mindfulness exercises, analogous to paying attention to your breathing during a strenuous ascent. You can maintain your composure and attention during the shift by using deep breathing techniques or meditation.

Keep an Eye on Your Body: Notice your physical and mental well-being. Individuals may experience ketosis in different ways, so pay attention to your body's cues. Similar to how a cyclist modifies their speed and gears, you may need to make little tweaks to your routine depending on how you're feeling.

Plan Your Meals Wisely: If you're on an intermittent fasting regimen, you might want to think about scheduling your nighttime meals. This can lessen your chance of experiencing hunger pains and help you make better use of your energy throughout the day.

Wrapping Up for Days 2-3

The second and third days of your fast are crucial. One major benefit of your fasting experience is that your body is growing more adept at burning fat for energy. It feels like you've reached the top of a difficult hill on your bike trip, and now you can enjoy the thrilling descent.

You may help your body enter ketosis by actively supporting it with mindfulness exercises, water retention, and light exercise. As you continue to use your body's fat reserves for energy, this phase will prepare you for the days ahead and help you reach your fasting objectives.

---Day 4-5---

The Stage of Adaptation

Days 4 and 5 are similar to learning your pace on a protracted bike trip or walk. Your body has become used to the fasting regimen, and you are feeling more energized and less hungry.

Here are some realistic things to think about and things to anticipate when going through this phase:

Knowing the Adaptation Phase and How Your Body Adjusts

Your body has completely acclimated to the fasting regimen by Days 4-5. It's like when your muscles adjust to a strenuous trek or when your bike finds its rhythm after a lengthy ride. Your energy levels are stable, and you're not feeling as hungry as before. It indicates that your body has successfully adapted to using fat that has been stored as fuel.

Physical Modifications: Greater Comfort and Vigor

Your appetite might have greatly decreased, much like the discomfort that hikers experience wearing off as they get used to the terrain. You will probably feel energized, like a rider finding their cadence on a beautiful, level bike ride. The goal of this phase is to feel more at ease and energized during your fasting regimen.

Things to Do on Days 4-5

Moderate Exercise: You might want to think about doing some moderate exercise now that your energy levels are more steady. This is similar to going for a leisurely bike ride or stroll. Choose exercises like cycling, gentle jogging, or brisk walking. Exercise can help you burn fat and improve your overall feeling of well-being.

Meal Planning: Now that you're not as hungry, it's a good idea to arrange your meals for the next few days. Make sure the food you choose to eat within your eating windows supports your fasting objectives. It's similar to planning your path for the remainder of your bike trip or trek.

Remain Hydrated: Make staying hydrated a priority. In addition to being necessary for your general health, water can assist you in controlling any residual little hunger cues.

Reflection and mindfulness: Give your journey some thought. Throughout the fasting process, mindfulness can support you in staying in touch with your objectives and feelings, much like a tranquil break during a hike or bike ride.

Support Network: Continue to interact with your network of support. Tell your friends, family, and online community about your experiences. It's similar to talking and exchanging voyage tales with other hikers or bikers.

Wrapping up Days 4-5

The first four and fifth days of your fast are the most exhilarating. Your body has been accustomed to the fasting regimen, which makes it more comfortable and energy-saving. It's like when you get your groove on a long bike ride or walk and the hardships at the beginning become easier to handle.

You will continue to thrive during this adaption phase if you plan your meals carefully, remain hydrated, practice mindfulness, and maintain connections with your support network in addition to moderate exercise. Your body will get more comfortable and energetic as you go along, which will strengthen your will to complete the 30-day fast and help you get closer to your wellness objectives.

CHAPTER 9

THE STAGE OF FAT BURNING

---Day 6---

Mark Advancements and Schedule Meals

You've accomplished a significant turning point in your fasting journey on Day 6. It's a day to celebrate your accomplishments and lay the groundwork for future success.

1. Honor Your Accomplishments:

In the morning, take time to celebrate your accomplishments to date. Now that you've successfully finished your five days of fasting, give it some thought. This can help you become more motivated and create a good mood for the rest of the day

Think about keeping a notebook to document your thoughts, emotions, and physical changes during the previous five days. This notebook can be an invaluable tool for tracking your fasting experience and offering support as you go.

2. Plan Meals High in Nutrients:

It's critical to schedule meals that will help you achieve your fasting objectives as your eating window draws closer. Eating foods high in nutrients will give you energy, vital vitamins, and minerals without interfering with your fat-burning phase.

Choose a well-balanced dinner that consists of:

- Lean proteins: Tofu, salmon, poultry, and turkey are a few examples.

An abundance of vegetables: Broccoli, spinach, kale, bell peppers, and other colorful, non-starchy vegetables are great options.

- Healthy fats: Include foods like almonds, avocados, and olive oil that are high in healthy fats.

Whole grains (optional): Use whole grains like brown rice or quinoa if you decide to include grains.

3. Hydration

Pour yourself a glass of water before you start eating. Water can help you feel more satiated before your meal, and staying hydrated is vital throughout your fasting journey.

If you find that black coffee or herbal teas help you control your desires and hunger, then go ahead and enjoy them. Just be aware of any calories or extra sweets in your drinks.

4. Exercise Intentional Eating

Eat mindfully when you are eating. This entails paying attention to your body's signals of hunger and fullness as well as concentrating on the sensory experience of eating.

Eat carefully, chewing and enjoying every bite. By using this method, you can avoid overindulging and better appreciate the tastes and textures of your food.

5. Monitoring Development

Keep an eye on your development both during and after your meal. How do you feel, emotionally and physically? Do you still feel hungry, or are you satisfied? These observations can help you make better dietary decisions in the future.

To sum up, Day 6 is a time to recognize your accomplishments and establish the tone for the remainder of your fast. You can make sure that you're feeding your body and maintaining your fat-burning phase at the same time by organizing meals that are high in nutrients, engaging in mindful eating, and drinking enough water. This strategy will assist you in staying on course to achieve your fasting objectives.

It is crucial to incorporate moderate activity and careful nutrition during Days 7-8 of your fasting journey. The following is a summary of the kinds of food and exercise that can be helpful on certain days:

--- Day 7 - 8 ---

Mindful Eating and Moderate Exercise

1. Moderate Workout:

Moderate exercise can improve your general health and speed up the process of burning fat. Consider the following exercise options:

Walking at a Quick Pace: This is a great way to get some moderate exercise in. It's a terrific technique to raise your heart rate and is low-impact and easily accessible. On these days, try to get in a 30-minute stroll.

Cycling: Taking a leisurely ride on a bicycle can be a fun and productive exercise if you have access to one. You can be active throughout your fast by going on walks in your neighborhood or along adjacent trails.

Yoga: Yoga is a great method to incorporate awareness into physical activity. Strength, balance, and flexibility can all be enhanced by it. Think about adding a 20–30 minute yoga class to your fasting regimen.

Light Jogging: If you're comfortable running, jogging for 20 to 30 minutes at a moderate pace will give your heart a good workout without being too taxing.

2. Conscious Eating

Pay attention to mindful eating on Days 7-8 during your eating windows. This method invites you to become aware of the sensory aspects of eating and to follow your body's signals of hunger and fullness. These are a few dietary guidelines:

- Lean Proteins: Consume foods high in lean protein, such as fish, turkey, or grilled chicken. These proteins help maintain muscle mass in addition to being fulfilling.

- Plenty of Vegetables: Include a range of vibrant, non-starchy veggies in your meals. Broccoli, spinach, kale, and bell peppers are examples of nutrient-dense, high-fiber foods that can make you feel full.

Add sources of good fats, such as almonds, avocados, and olive oil. These fats support general health and are satisfying.

- Whole Grains (Optional): Choose whole grains such as brown rice, quinoa, or whole wheat pasta if you decide to include grains. Comprising complex carbs, whole grains can offer prolonged energy.

- Hydration: Keep sipping water during your meal. Maintaining adequate hydration can aid in digestion and increase feelings of fullness.

Eat mindfully, chew your meal slowly, and pay attention to your body's signals of hunger and fullness with each bite. Overeating can be avoided and a healthy connection with food can be fostered through mindful eating.

In conclusion, try moderate exercise on Days 7-8, such as mild running, cycling, yoga, or brisk walking. Choose a variety of vegetables, lean proteins, healthy fats, and whole grains if you'd like. Make mindful eating a priority and make sure you're giving your body what it needs to support your fasting objectives.

---Day 9---

Fasting Techniques

A common method of fasting that alternates between eating and fasting times is called intermittent fasting. It may be a versatile and useful strategy to help you achieve your fasting objectives.

Some strategies for intermittent fasting to think about are as follows:

1. The 16/8 Method entails limiting your eating window to eight hours and fasting for sixteen hours. For instance, you may decide to fast from 8:00 PM to 12:00 PM the following day and eat between 12:00 PM and 8:00 PM on that day. You can drink black coffee, herbal tea, or water throughout the fasting period without consuming a substantial amount of calories.

Practical Aspect: Schedule your meals for when it works best with your schedule. You can change the time if you would rather have breakfast. On fasting days, it's critical to stick to your selected 8-hour eating window consistently.

2. The 5:2 Method: This strategy involves eating regularly for five days a week and drastically cutting calories (around 500–600) on the two non-consecutive days that are left. You can spread out your calorie intake during your fasting days with modest meals or snacks.

Practical Aspect: Select the two non-contiguous fasting days that are most convenient for you. To stay within the calorie limit on these days, prepare straightforward, low-calorie meals. To stay hydrated, make sure you consume lots of water.

3. Eat-Stop-Eat: This approach calls for one or two 24-hour fasts every week. You might, for instance, finish dinner at 7:00 PM and skip breakfast the next day. You only drink non-caloric beverages like tea or water when you're fasting.

Practical Aspect: Choose the days for the 24-hour fast that fit into your schedule. Keep yourself occupied and involved in activities to help block off hunger signs. During the fasting phase, stay well-hydrated.

4. Alternate-Day Fasting: This method involves switching between regular eating days and fasting days. You either eat nothing at all or very little (around 500 calories) during fasting days. You eat as normal on days when you are supposed to.

Practical Aspect: Schedule your meals and fasting periods ahead of time. Have a plan for either a full fast or low-calorie meal on fasting days. On eating days, think about consuming meals that are high in nutrients to enhance your general nutrition.

5. Warrior Diet: This diet calls for a single, substantial meal to be had during a 4-hour window in the evening after a 20-hour fast. During the fasting phase, you may have small portions of raw fruits and vegetables.

Practical Aspect: To meet your nutritional demands, plan your huge dinner to contain a combination of vegetables, healthy fats, and protein. To maximize the time you have for eating, concentrate on nutrient-rich foods.

Select an intermittent fasting technique that fits your preferences and way of life when you try it. Maintaining a healthy, well-balanced diet during your eating windows is crucial. Observe your body's signals of hunger and fullness and modify your fasting schedule accordingly. Recall that during times of fasting, maintaining adequate hydration is essential.

---Day 10---

Evaluate Results and Make Plans

On the tenth day of your fast, the emphasis is on reviewing your development and establishing new objectives. Monitoring your progress and maintaining the direction of your fasting journey is a crucial step

1. Assess Your Development

Consider your past experiences as you begin your day. Think about the following elements:

Physical Changes: Have you observed any physical changes in your body, such as a decrease in weight, an increase in energy, or better mental clarity?

Emotional Health: What emotional state have you been in for the last ten days? Have you encountered any difficulties with motivation or mood, or have you felt a feeling of accomplishment?

Hunger and Appetite: Observe the changes in your hunger and appetite. Have your eating patterns or urges changed at all?

General Well-Being: Evaluate your general state of health and happiness. Do you feel more in charge of your well-being and health now?

2. Record Your Results

Write down your observations in a journal or other document. Throughout your fasting journey, keeping a journal of your feelings and progress can keep you motivated and offer insightful information for the future.

3. Establish New Objectives

It's time to make fresh plans for the next stage of your fasting adventure based on your assessment. When defining your objectives, take into account the following:

Specificity: Clearly state your objectives. Rather than stating, "I want to lose weight," be more specific about the amount of weight you want to drop or the other health benefits you want to achieve.

Measurability: Establish quantifiable objectives. This enables you to monitor your development and recognize your accomplishments. If your objective is to lose weight, for example, specify how many pounds or kilos you want to shed.

Realistic Objectives: Make sure your objectives are doable and attainable in a fair amount of time. Instead of setting yourself up for failure, focus on your success.

Timeline: Decide on a deadline for your objectives. Determine when you hope to accomplish them. This could be a longer-term objective or after your 30-day fast.

Flexibility: Be willing to modify your objectives as necessary. Since your body's reaction to fasting can differ, it's critical to be adaptable and change your objectives as needed.

4. Put Your General Health First

Setting objectives for weight loss or other particular results is important, but don't forget to give your general health and well-being priority. Think about establishing objectives for increased mental clarity, better sleep, more energy, and long-term health maintenance.

5. Seek Assistance and Responsibility

Inform your support network—friends, family, or an online community—of your objectives. Others' support and accountability can be quite helpful in assisting you in reaching your goals.

6. Make a plan of action.

After you've determined your objectives, draft a workable action plan. Ascertain the actions and approaches you must take to achieve your objectives. This can entail tweaking your fasting regimen, adding particular workouts, or improving the meals you choose to eat.

7. Remain Dedicated

Give your aims your all attention and perseverance. Maintaining consistency is essential to the success of your fasting journey. As you proceed, remember your objectives and make decisions that support them.

Day 10 becomes a crucial day in your fasting journey when you evaluate your progress, make new goals, and create a strong action plan. It's a chance to restate your goals and keep working toward your objectives, which could include losing weight, getting healthier, or improving your overall well-being.

CHAPTER 10

UNLOCKING YOUR POTENTIAL FOR ENERGY

---Day 11---

Embrace Fasting Energy

At this stage of your fasting adventure, your body has evolved to use stored fat for energy efficiently. This is like a well-maintained car running on high-quality gasoline, ensuring a smooth and dynamic ride. Here's an additional explanation of what to do on Day 11:

1. Feel the Energy: On Day 11, you'll likely feel a rise in your energy levels. Your body is using its energy reserves to produce this, much way an efficient car uses its fuel. Embrace this energy and embrace the lightness and vibrancy it gives.

2. Active endeavors: Use this increased vitality to engage in active endeavors. Much like a car's engine functioning smoothly, your body is poised for action and productivity. Consider these activities:

Morning Exercise: Begin your day with a brisk morning stroll or a quick training session. This might help you feel revitalized and establish a positive tone for the day.

Productive chores: Dedicate time to accomplish chores or initiatives that need energy and focus. Much like a car efficiently covers kilometers, you can make tremendous progress in your regular activities.

3. Remain Hydrated: Make staying hydrated a priority. Proper hydration improves your body's energy levels and overall well-being. It's like ensuring your automobile has adequate coolant to prevent overheating after a lengthy ride.

4. Mindful Reflection: Take opportunities during the day to reflect on your energy levels and how they affect your mood and productivity. Much like savoring the scenery on a road trip, mindfulness can help you stay in the present and make the most of your energies.

5. Keep a Positive mentality: Maintain a positive mentality regarding your fasting experience. Acknowledge the energy spike as a positive indicator of improvement. Just like a well-fueled car works smoothly, your well-nourished body can function properly.

In summary, Day 11 is a day to fully appreciate the energy that your body is generating via fasting. Enjoy the sense of vitality and use it to engage in active pursuits and productive activities. Staying hydrated, practicing mindfulness, and maintaining a positive mindset can help you make the most of this energy and continue your journey towards your fasting goals.

---Day 12---

Balanced Nutrition

On Day 12, the focus is on maintaining balanced nutrition, which entails ensuring that your meals provide a mix of critical nutrients. Just like a broad selection of tunes can enrich a road trip, diversified and balanced food is crucial to supporting your fasting journey. Here's something to consider:

1. Lean Proteins: Include sources of lean protein in your meals. These can contain options like:

Grilled chicken breast

Turkey

Fish (such as salmon or tilapia)

Tofu or tempeh for plant-based protein

2. Plenty of Vegetables: Include a range of vibrant, non-starchy veggies in your meals. These are rich in vitamins, minerals, and fiber. Some instances include:

Broccoli

Spinach

Kale

Bell peppers

Tomatoes

Zucchini

Asparagus

3. Healthy Fats: Include sources of healthy fats to promote your general well-being. These can include:

Avocado

Olive oil

Nuts (such as almonds, walnuts, or cashews)

Seeds (such as chia seeds or flaxseeds)

4. Whole Grains (Optional): If you prefer to incorporate grains in your meals, choose for whole grains, which are rich in fiber and give lasting energy. Examples of entire grains include:

Quinoa

Brown rice

Whole wheat pasta

Oats

5. Portion Control: Be cautious of portion proportions to ensure that you're not overeating. This is analogous to selecting the correct music for your playlist to ensure a balanced and entertaining experience.

6. Hydration: Continue to be well-hydrated by drinking water throughout the day. Proper hydration improves digestion and helps manage appetite.

7. Balanced Flavors: Experiment with herbs and spices to enhance the flavors of your dishes. This might make your balanced nutrition plan more pleasurable and rewarding.

8. Meal Timing: Consider when you're eating during your meal window. Ensure that your meals are spread out sufficiently to control hunger and energy levels successfully.

In summary, Day 12 is about prioritizing balanced nutrition in your meals. Focus on ingesting lean proteins, an array of veggies, healthy fats, and whole grains if desired. Ensure portion control, remain hydrated, and use herbs and spices to make delectable meals. By maintaining a balanced and nutritious diet, you'll continue to support your fasting journey and keep your energy levels stable.

---Day 13---

Try a New Exercise

On Day 13, the idea is to try a new workout to keep your fitness program intriguing and your body engaged. Here are some suggestions for the type of workout you can explore

1. Yoga: Consider attempting yoga if you haven't previously. Yoga offers a wide range of styles, from easy and meditative to more rigorous and physically demanding. It's good for improving flexibility, balance, and total body awareness.

2. Pilates: Pilates is a low-impact exercise that focuses on core strength, flexibility, and posture. It's a terrific technique to target specific muscle groups and improve your general body alignment.

3. Dance: Dancing can be a fun and effective method to begin active. You can attempt other dance genres like hip-hop, salsa, or even ballet. Dancing not only provides a cardiovascular workout but also improves coordination.

4. Bodyweight workouts: Explore bodyweight workouts like calisthenics. This comprises motions such as push-ups, squats, lunges, and planks. Bodyweight workouts are versatile and may be tailored to different fitness levels.

5. Swimming: If you have access to a pool, swimming is a terrific full-body workout. It's low-impact, making it suited for varied fitness levels. Swimming can improve cardiovascular health and muscle strength.

6. Hiking: If you prefer spending time outdoors, hiking is a terrific option. It allows you to connect with nature while offering a terrific cardiovascular workout. Look for hiking routes in your neighborhood and choose one that matches your fitness level.

7. High-Intensity Interval Training (HIIT): HIIT workouts involve short bursts of high-intensity activity followed by brief recovery periods. They can be particularly helpful for enhancing cardiovascular fitness and burning calories.

8. Resistance Training: If you haven't tried resistance training, consider utilizing resistance bands or weights to target certain muscle regions. Resistance training can assist in developing muscle strength and tone.

9. Group Fitness Courses: Many gyms and fitness studios offer group fitness courses such as spinning, Zumba, or circuit training. Joining a class can provide a social aspect to your workout and inspire.

10. Outdoor Sports: Depending on your preferences, you can try outdoor sports like tennis, basketball, or even Frisbee. These sports are not only physically challenging but also pleasurable.

The idea is to find a workout that corresponds with your interests and fitness level. Trying a new activity keeps your routine fresh and might prevent monotony. It also challenges multiple muscle groups, leading to a well-rounded training routine. Remember to start gently, especially if the exercise is new to you, and stress safety and appropriate form.

---Day 14---

Practice Mindfulness

1. Find a peaceful area: Start by choosing a peaceful and comfortable area where you won't be easily distracted. This spot could be at your home, a park, or simply a pleasant corner in a coffee shop.

2. Comfortable Posture: Sit in a comfortable position. You can sit on a chair with your feet flat on the ground or cross-legged on the floor. The idea is to have a straight, yet comfortable posture.

3. Focus on Your Breath: Close your eyes if you feel comfortable doing so, and direct your attention to your breath. Observe your breath as it flows in and out. Pay attention to the sensation of the breath entering and leaving your body.

4. Be Present: As you focus on your breath, be fully present in the moment. If your mind starts to wander or thoughts come, recognize them without judgment and gently guide your focus back to your breath.

5. Body Scan: Take a few moments to mentally scan your body. Start at your toes and work your way up to the top of your head. Notice any places of tension or discomfort and let them relax.

6. Acceptance: Practice self-acceptance and self-compassion. Just as you wouldn't criticize the scenery on a road trip, stop criticizing your ideas, feelings, or body experiences. Let them be as they are without assigning labels or judgment.

7. Breath Awareness: Return your attention to your breath. You can count your breaths or simply observe them. Breathing in, count "one." Breathing out, count "two." Continue until you reach ten and then start over.

8. Mindful Eating: You may also include mindfulness in your meals. Savor each bite, paying attention to the flavors, textures, and how the meal makes you feel. Eat slowly and chew your food completely.

9. Gratitude: Take a minute to think about what you're grateful for. Gratitude is a vital element of mindfulness and can help cultivate a happy mentality.

10. Daily Practice: Mindfulness is most effective when practiced daily. Consider introducing small mindfulness sessions into your everyday routine, whether it's in the morning, during breaks, or before bed.

Mindfulness is a crucial technique for preserving emotional balance and increasing general well-being during your fasting journey. It can help you stay in the present moment, reduce stress, and boost your mental clarity. By practicing mindfulness, you're nurturing both your body and mind while you strive towards your fasting goals.

---Day 15---

Reconnect with Your Goals

1. Reflection on Your Journey:

Begin the day by reflecting on your journey so far. Consider the goals you established when you started your fasting journey. Reflect on the initial motivations and reasons that encouraged you to embark on this journey

2. Assess Your Development

Assess your progress since you started your fasting journey. Think about the following elements:

Physical Changes: Have you observed any physical changes in your body, such as a decrease in weight, an increase in energy, or better mental clarity?

Emotional Well-Being: How have you felt emotionally during the previous 15 days? Have you encountered any difficulties with motivation or mood, or have you felt a feeling of accomplishment?

Hunger and Appetite: Observe the changes in your hunger and appetite. Have your eating patterns or urges changed at all?

General Well-Being: Evaluate your general state of health and happiness. Do you feel more in charge of your well-being and health now?

3. Record Your Results:

Write down your observations in a journal or other document. Throughout your fasting journey, keeping a journal of your feelings and progress can keep you motivated and offer insightful information for the future.

4. Revisit Your Goals:

Revisit the goals you set at the beginning of your fasting adventure. Are these goals still significant to you?

Are there any adjustments you'd like to make?

5. Setting New Goals:

Based on your assessment and reflections, select new goals for the next chapter of your fasting adventure. When defining your objectives, take into account the following:

Specificity: Clearly state your objectives. Rather than stating, "I want to lose weight," be more specific about the amount of weight you want to drop or the other health benefits you want to achieve.

Measurability: Establish quantifiable objectives. This enables you to monitor your development and recognize your accomplishments. If your objective is to lose weight, for example, specify how many pounds or kilos you want to shed.

Realistic Objectives: Make sure your objectives are doable and attainable in a fair amount of time. Instead of setting yourself up for failure, focus on your success.

Timeline: Decide on a deadline for your objectives. Determine when you hope to accomplish them. This could be a longer-term objective or after your 30-day fast.

Flexibility: Be willing to modify your objectives as necessary. Since your body's reaction to fasting can differ, it's critical to be adaptable and change your objectives as needed.

6. Share Your Goals:

Inform your support network—friends, family, or an online community—of your objectives. Others' support and accountability can be quite helpful in assisting you in reaching your goals.

7. Make a plan of action.

Once you've identified your new goals, build a practical action plan. Ascertain the actions and approaches you must take to achieve your objectives. This can entail tweaking your fasting regimen, adding particular workouts, or improving the meals you choose to eat.

8. Remain Dedicated:

Give your aims your all attention and perseverance. Maintaining consistency is essential to the success of your fasting journey. As you proceed, remember your objectives and make decisions that support them.

By reconnecting with your goals, analyzing your success, and creating new targets, Day 15 becomes a critical stage in your fasting journey. It's a chance to restate your goals and keep working toward your objectives, which could include losing weight, getting healthier, or improving your overall well-being.

143

CHAPTER 11

WELLNESS AND HORMONE BALANCE

---Day 16---

Hormone Regulation

Hormone control is a crucial element of overall health, and fasting can play a significant role in maintaining or restoring equilibrium. Here's a full description of the concept:

1. Insulin Sensitivity: Fasting can boost insulin sensitivity, which is critical for managing blood sugar levels. When you fast, your body becomes more efficient at using insulin to move glucose into cells for energy. This is like fine-tuning a car's engine to enhance fuel economy.

2. Ghrelin and Leptin: Fasting can impact hormones like ghrelin and leptin, which are crucial for hunger regulation. Ghrelin, frequently termed the "hunger hormone," increases when your stomach is empty and drops after you've eaten. Leptin, known as the "satiety hormone," sends fullness to your brain. Fasting can help reset these hormones, making it easier to manage your appetite and food consumption.

3. Human Growth Hormone (HGH): Fasting can boost the secretion of human growth hormone (HGH), which plays a key role in growth, metabolism, and general health. HGH helps maintain lean body mass and aids fat metabolism. It's like turning up the motor of your body's repair and rejuvenation processes.

4. Cortisol Management: Fasting can help control cortisol, the body's principal stress hormone. Chronic stress can lead to abnormalities in cortisol levels, impacting many body systems. Fasting and stress reduction practices can help control cortisol, leading to improved hormonal balance.

5. Hormone Balance for Weight Management: Achieving hormonal balance through fasting might be essential in weight management. When hormones like insulin and leptin are in check, it becomes simpler to control your appetite, manage body weight, and prevent overeating.

6. Long-Term Health Benefits: Maintaining hormonal balance through fasting is not only advantageous in the short term but also adds to long-term health. Balanced hormones can minimize the incidence of metabolic illnesses like diabetes and enhance general wellness.

7. Fasting tactics: On this day, you'll investigate numerous fasting tactics that can be utilized to optimize hormone balance. This encompasses approaches such as intermittent fasting, extended fasting, and time-restricted eating.

Remember that hormone control is a complex process, and the influence of fasting might differ from person to person. It's vital to listen to your body and consult with a healthcare practitioner if you have specific concerns about your hormones or any pre-existing health disorders. Fasting, when done appropriately and carefully, maybe a helpful tool for reaching hormonal balance and supporting your overall health and wellness.

---Day 17---

Stress Management

1. Mindfulness Meditation: Practice mindfulness meditation to become more aware of the present moment. Mindfulness helps you manage stress by teaching your mind to focus on the here and now, eliminating worries about the past or future.

2. Deep Breathing Exercises: Deep breathing techniques, such as diaphragmatic breathing, can assist in activating the body's relaxation response. Take slow, deep breaths to calm your anxious system.

3. Progressive Muscle Relaxation: This procedure involves tensing and then relaxing specific muscle groups in your body. It's a great approach to alleviate bodily tension and reduce stress.

4. Yoga: Yoga combines physical postures, breathing exercises, and meditation to increase flexibility and relieve stress. It's a fantastic practice for both physical and mental well-being.

5. Regular Exercise: Engaging in regular physical activity can help manage stress by generating endorphins, the body's natural mood boosters. Whether it's a brisk stroll, jogging, or any other sort of exercise, it can reduce stress and enhance your general mood.

6. Time Management: Effective time management can help you reduce stress by allowing you to prioritize chores and avoid feeling overwhelmed. Use tactics like to-do lists and scheduling to keep organized.

7. Conscious Eating: Pay attention to what you eat during your fasting journey. Enjoy your meals carefully, appreciating each bite. This can alleviate tension and aid digestion.

8. Journaling: Keeping a journal can be a powerful stress management strategy. Write down your thoughts and feelings to get insight into your pressures and build ways to deal with them.

9. Seek Support: Don't hesitate to seek out friends, family, or a therapist for help. Talking about your concerns and feelings can give relief and helpful insights.

10. Engage in Relaxing Activities: Participate in activities that you find calming, such as reading, listening to music, having a hot bath, or spending time in nature.

11. Limit Stimulants: Limit your usage of stimulants like caffeine and nicotine, which can raise tension and anxiety.

12. Sleep Hygiene: Prioritize sound sleep by developing a nighttime routine and ensuring a pleasant sleep environment. Adequate rest is vital for stress management.

13. Laughter & Humor: Incorporate comedy into your daily lives. Laughter may be an effective stress reliever, producing endorphins and enhancing your mood.

14. Self-Compassion: Be gentle and sympathetic to yourself. Recognize that it's good to experience periods of tension, and don't be too hard on yourself.

Remember that different stress management approaches work well for different people. Experiment with these tactics to determine what connects with you. Combining several of these approaches can provide a complete approach to stress management, ensuring you're more ready to handle stress during your fasting journey and in your regular life.

---Day 18---

Sleep and Hormones - Practical Aspects

Day 18, which is all about the connection between sleep and hormones during your fasting journey. Quality sleep is vital for hormone balance and overall well-being. Here's how to practically utilize this knowledge:

Establish a Consistent Sleep routine: Stick to a regular sleep routine by going to bed and waking up at the same times each day, even on weekends. This constancy helps control your body's internal clock, encouraging hormone balance.

Create a Relaxing nighttime ritual: Develop a peaceful nighttime ritual to communicate to your body that it's time to wind down. Activities like reading, having a warm bath, or practicing relaxation techniques help prepare you for a good night's sleep.

Optimize Your Sleep Environment: Ensure your sleep environment is conducive to quality rest. This implies a comfy mattress and pillows, a cool room temperature, and little noise and light interruptions.

Limit Screen Time Before Bed: The blue light emitted by screens might interrupt your sleep-wake cycle. Try to avoid screens (phones, computers, TVs) at least an hour before bedtime. If you must use screens, consider utilizing blue light filters.

Avoid Heavy Meals and Caffeine Late in the Day: Large, heavy meals close to bedtime might impair sleep. Similarly, coffee should be avoided in the afternoon and evening, as it can interfere with your ability to fall asleep.

Be Hydrated: While it's crucial to be hydrated, try to restrict your fluid intake in the hours preceding bedtime to prevent nightly awakenings for toilet excursions.

Regular Exercise: Engage in regular physical activity, but try to complete your exercise program at least a couple of hours before bedtime. Exercise can promote better sleep, but doing it too close to bedtime may have the opposite impact.

Manage Stress: Incorporate stress management strategies, such as mindfulness meditation or deep breathing exercises, into your daily routine to reduce tension and anxiety, both of which can interfere with sleep.

Limit Naps: While short power naps can be refreshing, extended daytime naps might impair your overnight sleep. If you feel the desire to snooze, strive for a brief nap of 20-30 minutes.

Limit Alcohol: Avoid excessive alcohol consumption, especially in the evening. While alcohol may initially make you tired, it might lead to disordered sleep habits.

Careful Eating: During your fasting journey, be careful of when and what you eat. Avoid heavy meals too soon to bedtime, as they can induce discomfort and impact sleep quality.

Journaling: If you have racing thoughts or worries before bedtime, consider maintaining a notebook to jot down your concerns. This can help cleanse your mind and lessen worry.

By adding these practical factors into your daily routine, you can encourage better sleep and hormonal balance during your fasting journey. Quality sleep is crucial for general wellness, and it complements the favorable benefits of fasting on hormone control and well-being.

---Day 19---

Female Hormones - Impact and Adaptation

Day 19, which focuses on female hormones and how fasting can affect them. It's crucial to recognize these consequences and alter your fasting technique properly to enhance your general well-being

1. Menstrual Cycle: Fasting can alter the menstrual cycle in some women, particularly if they are already prone to irregular periods. It's vital to monitor your cycle and be prepared for potential changes.

2. Amenorrhea: In certain situations, prolonged fasting or excessive calorie restriction can lead to amenorrhea, the lack of menstruation. This is often a symptom that the body's hormone balance has been upset.

3. Adapted Fasting Approach: If you notice changes in your menstrual cycle or amenorrhea due to fasting, it's vital to alter your approach. Consider the following adjustments:

Less Restrictive Fasting: Opt for less restrictive fasting approaches, such as intermittent fasting, that allow for regular nutrient intake and limit the danger of hormone abnormalities.

Nutrient-Dense Eating: Focus on nutrient-dense, balanced meals to ensure you are supplying your body with important vitamins and minerals. This helps hormonal health.

Consult a Healthcare expert: If you encounter major menstrual abnormalities or amenorrhea, consult a healthcare expert. They can help assess your specific condition and provide advice on changing your fasting technique.

4. Hormone Balance: Hormone balance is vital for general wellness. Female hormones like estrogen, progesterone, and testosterone play a key part in different body activities. Ensure that fasting does not lead to hormonal abnormalities that harm your well-being.

5. Monitor Symptoms: Pay special attention to how fasting impacts your emotions, energy levels, and overall health. If you observe symptoms such as mood swings, exhaustion, or irregular periods, consider modifying your fasting method.

6. Stress Reduction: Implement stress reduction tactics as stress might exacerbate hormonal abnormalities. Practices like yoga, meditation, and deep breathing might be extremely useful.

7. Balanced Diet: Consume a well-balanced diet rich in critical nutrients, including protein, healthy fats, and a range of fruits and vegetables. This can help support hormone balance.

8. Consult with a Healthcare Professional: If you have specific concerns regarding the influence of fasting on your female hormones, speak with a healthcare expert who specializes in women's health. They can provide specialized guidance and monitor your progress.

9. Personalized Approach: Recognize that every woman's experience with fasting and its impact on hormones can be unique. It's vital to personalize your fasting method to your specific demands and responses.

10. Focus on Health and Well-Being: Ultimately, your fasting journey should prioritize your health and well-being. If you find that fasting is negatively affecting your hormones and your health, it's crucial to reassess your strategy or seek different approaches for accomplishing your wellness goals.

By knowing the potential influence of fasting on female hormones and making necessary adjustments to your strategy, you may better support your hormonal health and overall well-being. Listening to your body and getting professional help when necessary are essential elements in this process.

---Day 20---

Hormone Balance for Men - In Detail

1. Testosterone and Hormone Balance: Testosterone is the primary male sex hormone and plays a crucial role in various aspects of health, including muscle mass, bone density, energy levels, and mood. Fasting can influence testosterone levels in men.

2. Positive Effects on Testosterone: Some research suggests that intermittent fasting may lead to a temporary increase in testosterone levels. This can be seen as the body's adaptive response to promote energy and maintain muscle mass.

3.Potential Challenges: However, extreme or prolonged fasting and excessive calorie restriction can lead to lower testosterone levels. It's important to strike a balance between fasting and maintaining hormonal health.

4. Stress Management: Stress can influence hormonal balance. Incorporate stress management techniques such as mindfulness, meditation, and deep breathing to reduce the potential negative effects of stress on hormones.

5. Comprehensive Health Approach: It's essential to view your fasting journey as part of your broader health strategy. Consider your overall well-being and hormonal health as you progress through your fasting journey.

6. Listen to Your Body: Pay attention to how your body responds to fasting. Monitor any changes in energy, mood, and physical health. Adjust your fasting approach as needed to maintain balance.

7. Holistic Well-Being: Prioritize holistic well-being, which includes factors like nutrition, exercise, sleep, and stress management, in addition to your fasting approach. A well-rounded approach is vital for maintaining hormone balance and overall health.

8. Consult with Professionals: If you have specific concerns or health issues related to male hormones, consult with healthcare professionals who specialize in men's health and hormonal balance. They can offer expert guidance tailored to your needs.

**9.	Individualized	Approach:** Recognize that every man's experience with fasting and its effects on hormones can be unique. Tailor your fasting approach to your specific needs and responses.

By understanding the potential impact of fasting on male hormones, making appropriate adjustments to your approach, and focusing on holistic well-being, you can better support your hormone balance and overall health during your fasting journey. Listening to your body and seeking professional guidance when necessary are essential steps in this process.

CHAPTER 12

THE LINK BETWEEN MIND AND BODY

---Day 21---

Mindful Eating - Nourishing the Body and Soul

Mindful eating is an art that goes beyond merely satisfying your hunger;

it's about nurturing your body and soul. This practice encourages you to be fully present in the dining experience, much like savoring a symphony or the beauty of nature.

As you engage in mindful eating, you're asked to slow down and appreciate the flavors and textures of your food, savoring each bite as if it were a precious moment in time. You observe your body's cues of hunger and fullness, much like tuning in to your favorite music. Distractions are set aside, and you create a sacred space where you and your meal become the entire universe.

By embracing mindful eating, you develop a profound connection with the nourishment your food provides, much like an artist connecting with their canvas. It fosters a healthier relationship with food, reducing overeating and emotional eating. It's an act of gratitude, acknowledging the effort and resources that brought this meal to your table. Mindful eating is a powerful tool for enhancing your fasting journey, cultivating a harmonious connection between your body and the nourishment it receives, and fostering a deep appreciation for the gift of nourishment in your life.

---Day 22---

Focus on emotional eating awareness.

It's an opportunity to recognize the connection between our emotions and the way we eat. Emotional eating often involves turning to food as a way to cope with stress, sadness, or other feelings. By becoming aware of these patterns, we can begin to address them, finding healthier ways to manage our emotions and reduce reliance on food for comfort. This day encourages self-reflection, helping individuals understand the triggers that lead to emotional eating and empowering them to make more mindful food choices in response to their emotional well-being.

---Day 23---

Day 23 is dedicated to stress reduction techniques, essential for maintaining well-being during your fasting journey. Stress can affect both the mind and body. This day offers practical strategies to manage stress effectively, including mindfulness meditation, deep breathing exercises, yoga, and relaxation practices. These techniques aim to calm the mind, reduce anxiety, and promote a sense of inner peace. By incorporating stress reduction practices, individuals can better cope with the challenges of fasting, improve their overall mood, and create a more harmonious mind-body connection, ultimately enhancing their fasting experience and overall wellness.

---Day 24---

Day 24 explores the power of positive thinking in enhancing your fasting journey. Positive thoughts and attitudes can influence both mental and physical health. By adopting an optimistic mindset, focusing on gratitude, and using positive affirmations, individuals can improve their overall well-being. This positive approach can help manage stress, boost resilience, and enhance motivation, making it easier to maintain your fasting regimen. The power of positive thinking is akin to having a guiding light, helping you navigate challenges with a hopeful spirit, and ultimately leading to a more rewarding and successful fasting experience.

---Day 25---

This day emphasizes the significance of self-care and self-compassion in your fasting journey. Self-care involves taking time to nurture your physical and mental well-being, much like tending to a garden. It includes practices such as rest, relaxation, and activities that bring joy. Self-compassion means treating yourself with kindness, as you would a dear friend, and understanding that it's okay to have setbacks or difficulties. It's essential for maintaining a positive mind-body connection and helping you navigate the challenges of fasting with resilience. Self-care and self-compassion are like the gentle touch that soothes your soul and fosters a sense of balance during your fasting experience.

CHAPTER 13

ENJOYING YOUR BENEFITS

---Day 26---

Celebrate Achievements - A Moment of Triumph

Today marks a jubilant milestone in your fasting journey. It's a day to celebrate the remarkable achievements you've made along the way. Like crossing the finish line of a challenging race, it's a moment of triumph that deserves recognition and applause.

Take a step back and reflect on how far you've come. Acknowledge the discipline, dedication, and resilience you've displayed throughout your fasting journey. Consider the physical and mental transformations you've experienced, from improved energy levels to increased self-awareness.

Celebrate your newfound sense of self-control, healthier eating habits, and the profound connection you've forged between your mind and body. Much like receiving a well-deserved award, this is your time to bask in the glory of your accomplishments.

Share your joy with loved ones or simply revel in the satisfaction of reaching this pivotal moment. Your fasting journey is a testament to your determination, and today, it's fitting to raise your flag of victory and acknowledge the triumph you've achieved.

---Day 27---

Reflect on Transformation - The Art of Self-Discovery

As you near the end of your fasting journey, Day 27 is dedicated to introspection and reflection. It's a time to contemplate the profound transformation you've undergone, both internally and externally. This is akin to an artist stepping back to appreciate the masterpiece they've created.

Take a moment to marvel at the changes you've witnessed. Physically, you may have experienced weight loss, increased energy, or improved well-being. Emotionally and mentally, you've likely gained self-awareness, self-control, and a deeper connection to your body. Like a caterpillar emerging from its chrysalis as a butterfly, your transformation is a testament to your growth.

Reflect on the lessons you've learned, the challenges you've conquered, and the resilience you've displayed. This day encourages you to acknowledge your journey, much like a traveler pausing to admire the landscape they've crossed. Recognize that transformation is a continuous process, and as you reflect on the path behind you, you're also preparing for the road ahead.

---Day 28---

Setting Future Goals - Paving the Way Forward

On Day 28, you stand at the threshold of your fasting journey's conclusion, ready to embark on the next chapter of your well-being. This day is like an explorer charting a new course. It's an opportunity to set your future goals and intentions.

Consider how fasting has positively impacted your life, both physically and mentally. Now, look ahead and think about how you can maintain and build upon these gains. Are there specific health goals you wish to achieve or aspects of your well-being you'd like to focus on?

Much like a captain plotting a course, outline a plan for your health and wellness journey. Define clear, achievable goals, and establish a roadmap to guide you toward success. Whether it's maintaining a healthy fasting routine, incorporating regular exercise, or exploring new mindful practices, this is your opportunity to take charge of your future well-being.

By setting future goals, you're not merely concluding your fasting journey but launching into a future filled with health, vitality, and personal growth.

This day is a bridge to the exciting possibilities that lie ahead.

---Day 29---

Express Gratitude - The Heartfelt Thank You

On Day 29, you're invited to take a moment to express profound gratitude for the journey you've undertaken. Much like the warmth of the sun breaking through the clouds after a storm, this is your opportunity to let gratitude illuminate your path.

Acknowledge the countless blessings that have accompanied your fasting journey. Express your thankfulness for the positive changes in your physical and mental well-being. Recognize the strength and resilience that have emerged within you, akin to a dormant seed sprouting into a vibrant flower.

Extend gratitude to the people who have supported and encouraged you on this path, whether it's friends, family, or healthcare professionals. Like the hands that nurture a garden, their support has helped you thrive.

Appreciate the lessons learned and the wisdom gained throughout this journey. Gratitude is a bridge to inner peace and contentment, much like a serene lake reflecting the beauty of the surrounding landscape.

By expressing gratitude, you're embracing the joy of the present moment and creating a foundation for future well-being. This is your heartfelt thank you to the universe for the gift of health and self-discovery.

---Day 30---

Celebrate Your Fasting Journey - The Grand Finale

Day 30 marks the grand finale of your fasting journey, a celebration of your remarkable accomplishments and newfound well-being. It's like reaching the peak of a challenging mountain and taking a moment to savor the breathtaking view.

This day is a testament to your unwavering commitment, resilience, and the transformative power of fasting. It's a time to bask in the sense of accomplishment, much like a victorious athlete crossing the finish line.

Celebrate the physical and mental changes you've undergone, from increased energy levels to greater self-awareness. Revel in the improved relationship you've forged with food and the profound mind-body connection you've cultivated.

This is your day to share your achievements with loved ones, acknowledge the support you've received, and inspire others on their health journeys. It's like a grand feast of gratitude and joy, honoring the path you've traveled.

As you celebrate your fasting journey, remember that this isn't the end but a

Launchpad for your ongoing well-being. It's a moment to reflect on your accomplishments and set your sights on a future filled with health, vitality, and personal growth.

Celebrating your fasting journey on Day 30 is a significant and personal endeavor. Here are various ways you might choose to commemorate this achievement:

Reflective Journaling: Write down your feelings and observations about the whole fasting process in your journal. Keep a journal of the difficulties you overcame, the knowledge you gained, and the improvements you saw.

Gratitude Meditation: To show gratitude for the experience, the lessons learned, and the enhancements to your well-being, engage in a gratitude meditation. Think back on the help you've gotten and the inner power you've found.

Healthy Feast: To break your fast, prepare a special, nourishing meal. Concentrate on eating nutrient-dense foods that support your health objectives. This could serve as a metaphor for the conclusion of your fasting period.

Fitness Celebration: Do something physical that makes you happy, be it a vigorous walk, a yoga practice, or any other kind of exercise. Appreciate the newfound vigor and strength in your body.

Connect with Loved Ones: Tell those who have helped you along the way about your accomplishments. Their support has been invaluable, and sharing the celebration with them can add even more significance to the achievement.

Make New Objectives: Today, make new health-related objectives. Whether it's sticking to your fasting schedule, trying out new workouts, or adding mindfulness exercises, making plans for your ongoing well-being is a step in the right direction.

Give yourself a day of self-care to pamper yourself. Treating yourself to a spa treatment, a soothing bath, or just indulging in your favorite activities is a worthy celebration.

Record Your Journey: Put your journey into visual form by making a timeline or collage. Add images, quotations, and significant dates to provide a physical reminder of your achievements.

Recall that the purpose of the celebration is to honor and recognize all of your efforts, no matter how small. Select pursuits that you find meaningful and that support your objectives for well-being. This is the day you've worked so hard for, so the celebration you choose should honor the significance of your fasting journey

SECTION III

CHAPTER 14

BENEFITS OF FASTING

Adopting a long-term fasting lifestyle can have several positive effects on health. The following are a few possible long-term benefits:

Weight management: By encouraging fat-burning and consuming fewer calories, fasting can help people lose weight. Additionally, by increasing metabolic flexibility, it might support weight maintenance.

Enhanced Insulin Sensitivity: Research has connected fasting to enhanced insulin sensitivity, which lowers the long-term risk of type 2 diabetes. This may improve the body's capacity to successfully control blood sugar levels.

Enhanced Cellular Repair: When a person fasts, their body goes through a process known as autophagy, which helps them replace damaged cells with healthy ones. This may enhance the general longevity and health of cells.

Cardiovascular Health: By lowering blood pressure, cholesterol, and the risk of heart disease, prolonged fasting may have a beneficial effect on cardiovascular health.

Brain Health: Studies have shown that fasting has a positive impact on cognition, possibly lowering the risk of neurodegenerative diseases like Alzheimer's disease and improving brain function.

Longevity: Research indicates that fasting may affect aging-related variables, possibly leading to a longer and better life.

Inflammatory Response: Several illnesses are associated with chronic inflammation. Fasting may support the health of the immune system overall by reducing inflammation.

Cancer Prevention: Studies suggest that fasting may help prevent cancer by affecting processes like cell metabolism and autophagy, but more research is required in this area.

Gut Health: A balanced and diverse microbial environment is essential for healthy digestion and overall well-being, and fasting may have a positive impact on gut microbiota.

Hormone Regulation: Insulin and human growth hormone (HGH), two important hormones for metabolism and general health, can be affected by fasting.

While there is some scientific evidence to support these potential benefits, it's important to remember that everyone reacts differently to fasting. Seeking advice from a healthcare professional is advised before committing to long-term fasting, particularly for individuals who already have health conditions or concerns. Furthermore, it is critical for general health during non-fasting periods to incorporate a balanced and nutrient-rich diet.

CHAPTER 15

HONOURING YOUR 30-DAY FASTING COMPLETION

"Celebrating Your 30-Day Fasting Achievement" is a momentous occasion that signifies the end of a noteworthy journey toward better health and well-being. Here are specific ideas on how to commemorate this achievement:

1. Consider Your Journey:

Journaling: Give your 30-day fasting experience some thought. Keep a journal of the difficulties you overcome, the knowledge you gained, and the improvements you saw. You can document the mental and physical changes by keeping a journal.

2. Manifest Your Thanks:

Gratitude Practice: Express your appreciation for the trip and the work you've put into improving your health. Think about thanking yourself, and your loved ones for your support, and the process that helped you reach your objectives.

3. Share Your Achievement:

Celebrate with Others: Tell your loved ones or friends who have helped you about your accomplishments. Their support has probably been a major factor in your accomplishment. To share your experience, think about hosting a modest party or hosting an online celebration.

4. In-person Celebration:

Exercise: Take Advantage of Your Newfound Vitality and Energy by Exercising in Something You Enjoy. Whether it's a dance class, a trip through the outdoors, or your go-to workout, move your body in a way that makes you feel joyous.

5. wholesome feast

Prepare a delicious Meal: Have a nutritious and delicious meal to break your fast. To make a festive feast, think about combining a range of nutrient-dense foods and flavors. This could be a tasty, nutritious dinner that supports your health objectives. It is also well-balanced.

6. Thinking and Being Present:

Yoga or meditation: To honor the mental and emotional facets of your journey, partake in a mindful exercise like yoga or meditation. This enables you to find your core, celebrate your successes, and live in the now.

7. Establish New Objectives:

Evaluate and Make New Goals: Take advantage of this milestone to review your health objectives. For the next stage of your wellness journey, make new goals. Think about achieving both short- and long-term objectives that complement your overarching well-being vision.

8. Establish a Graphical Representation:

Vision Board or Collage: Using a vision board or collage, make a visual depiction of your quest. Add pictures, sayings, and symbols that symbolize your goals, accomplishments, and the transformations you've gone through.

9. Honor yourself with self-care:

Pampering Session: Have a day of self-care for yourself. Celebrate your accomplishment by taking care of your body and mind, whether that means scheduling a spa day, taking a soothing bath, or just spending time doing things you enjoy.

10. Show gratitude and happiness:

Celebrate with Joy: Express your happiness and appreciation for the accomplishment to the community that helped you along the way or on social media. Others may find inspiration and motivation in your road toward well-being.

Recall that the celebration needs to be in line with your principles and have meaning for you. It's a deeply personal and significant recognition of your accomplishments, and the celebrations you decide on should be appropriate for the importance of finishing the 30-day fast.

Finally, the completion of your 30-day fast signifies the start of a fresh dedication to your health as well as the conclusion of a life-changing experience. You've used perseverance, discipline, and self-discovery to your advantage throughout this project, and you came out on the other side feeling really accomplished. As you consider the changes in your body and mind, keep in mind that this path involves more than just giving up food; it's an all-encompassing acceptance of mindful living that nourishes the body and the spirit.

The knowledge gained—whether from conquering obstacles or relishing successes—is a first step toward long-term health. It's not just about the number of days; it's also about the moments that are treasured, routines that are rethought, and awareness that is awoken. Carry the gratitude torch going forward for your body's tenacity and the encouragement you received from others

This is only the beginning of a lifelong journey toward wellness; it is not the end. Celebrate your renewed energy as you enter the post-fasting phase and allow the ripple effects of your accomplishments to carry into the future. Stay in tune with your body, make conscious decisions, and never forget that your path to better health is a dynamic mosaic that changes with every decision you make. Accept the knowledge gained, celebrate your accomplishments, and look forward with an open heart and a body full of energy for the next phase of your journey toward wellness.

CHAPTER 16

FREQUENTLY ASKED QUESTIONS

Here are some frequently asked questions (FAQ) that individuals might have about a 30-day fasting journey, along with concise solutions:

1. Q: Can I exercise during fasting days?

A: Yes, moderate exercise is generally safe during fasting days. Listen to your body, choose activities you enjoy, and stay hydrated. If in doubt, consult a healthcare professional.

2. Q: What can I eat during non-fasting days?

A: Focus on nutrient-dense foods such as lean proteins, whole grains, fruits, and vegetables. Maintain a balanced diet to support overall health.

3. Q: Will fasting help me lose weight?

A: Fasting can contribute to weight loss by creating a caloric deficit. However, individual results vary. It's crucial to pair fasting with a balanced diet and lifestyle.

4. Q: How do I deal with cravings during fasting?

A: Stay hydrated, distract yourself with activities, and choose filling, nutritious foods during non-fasting periods. Cravings often subside with time.

5. Q: Is fasting suitable for everyone?

A: Fasting may not be suitable for certain medical conditions or specific individuals. Consult with a healthcare professional before starting any fasting regimen.

6. Q: Can I fast if I have diabetes?

A: Individuals with diabetes should consult their healthcare provider before fasting. Fasting can affect blood sugar levels, and careful monitoring is essential.

7. Q: What are the potential side effects of fasting?

A: Side effects may include fatigue, irritability, or headaches. These often improve as the body adjusts. If severe or persistent, consult a healthcare professional.

8. Q: How do I break my fast safely?

A: Break your fast with a balanced meal, starting with smaller portions and easy-to-digest foods. Avoid overeating and opt for nutrient-dense options.

9. Q: Can I continue fasting beyond 30 days?

A: Extended fasting may have risks. Consult a healthcare professional before considering prolonged fasting. Consider intermittent fasting for long-term health benefits.

CONNECT WITH ME

Thank you very much for taking the time to read this book. This is a wonderful friendship, and I appreciate your trust and consideration so much. If you found meaning in these pages, if they moved you or piqued your interest, I hope you'll continue your journey with me into the rest of my writings. The stories, lessons, and experiences that fill the pages of my other published books were written with all of my heart and soul and are just waiting to be discovered by you.

Each book is a carefully woven tapestry of myriad feelings, sage advice, and stories that anyone can relate to, and I write them with the sincere desire that they will move you. If you've enjoyed this trip, I hope you'll also take the time to explore my other writings. Thank you for being a part of this literary trip, and I look forward to connecting with you through the magic of words once again!!!

www.ingramcontent.com/pod-product-compliance
Lightning Source LLC
Chambersburg PA
CBHW050724260726
48661CB00001B/57